JACK FEELS

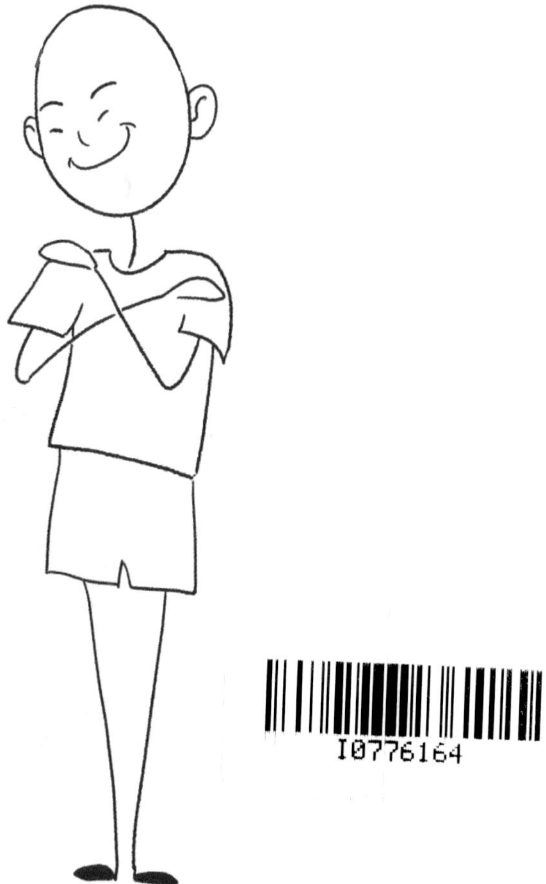

An Emotional Literacy Resource

For My Kids - Tommy & Angel

I love you more than Max loves to snuggle!
- Mom

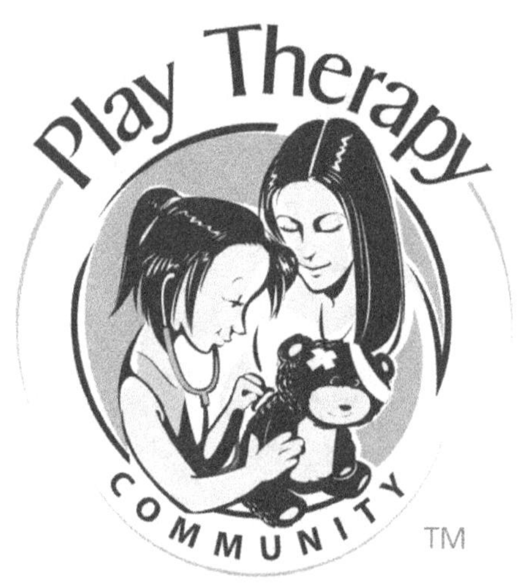

ISBN-13:
978-1976538544

ISBN-10:
1976538548

Duplication & Copyright

No part of this publication may be reproduced or transmitted in any form by any means without prior permission from the author.

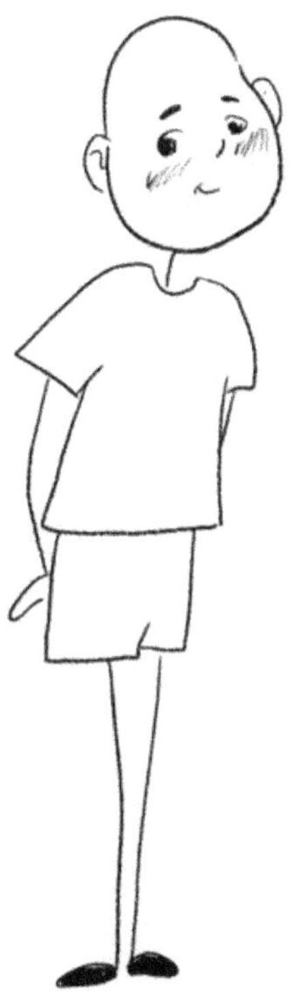# EMBARRASSED

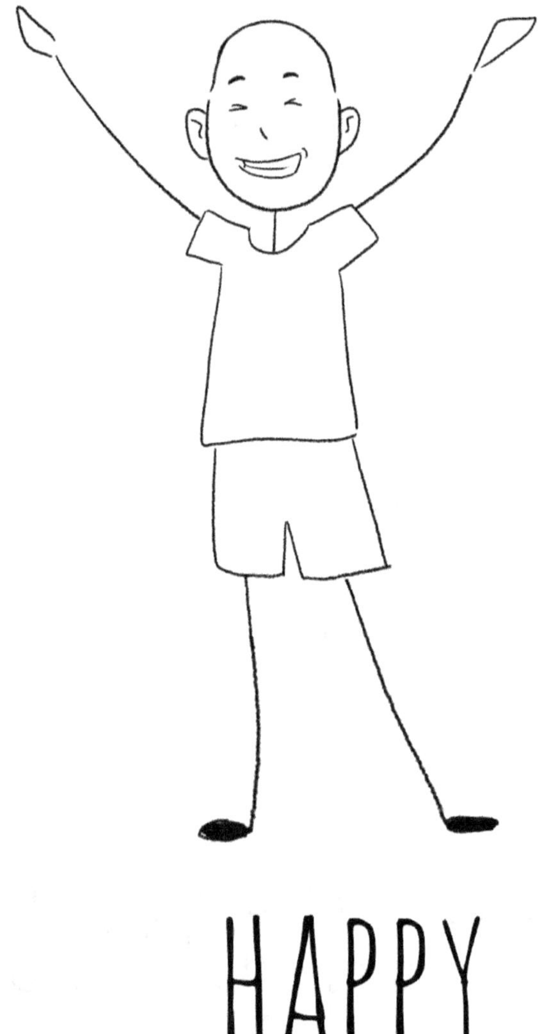

HAPPY

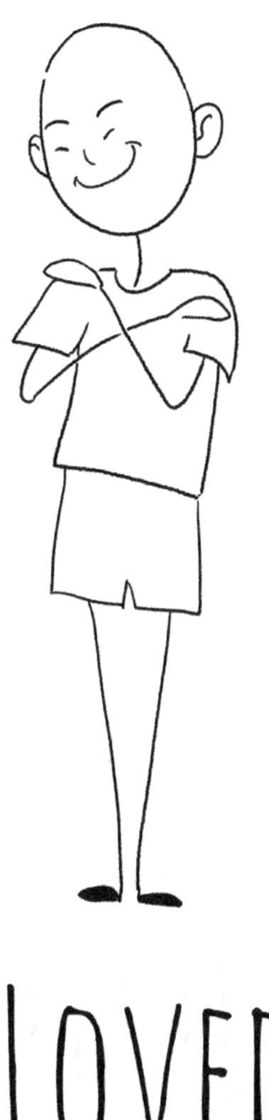

LOVED

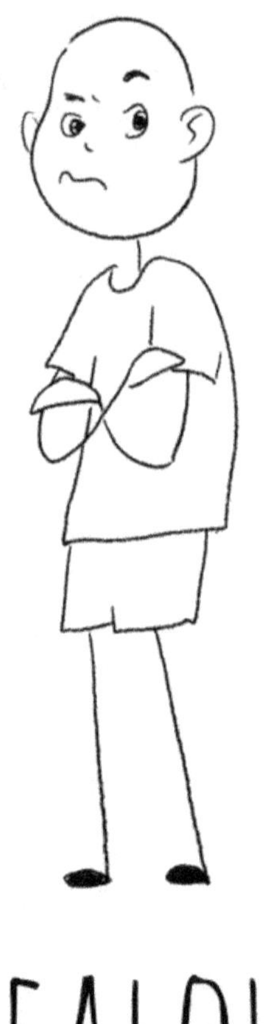

JEALOUS

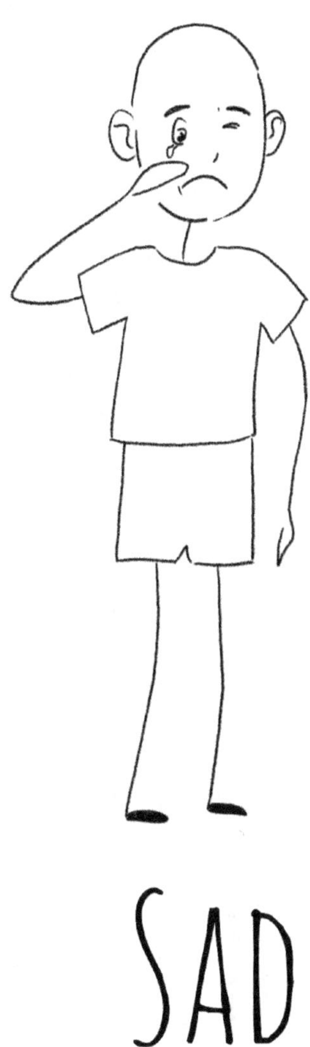

SAD

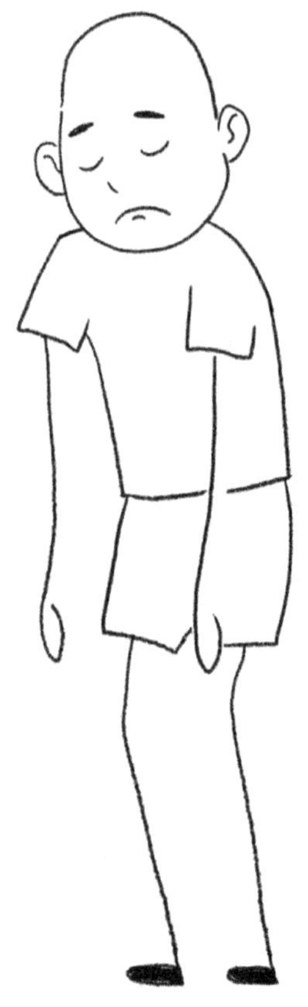

DISAPPOINTED

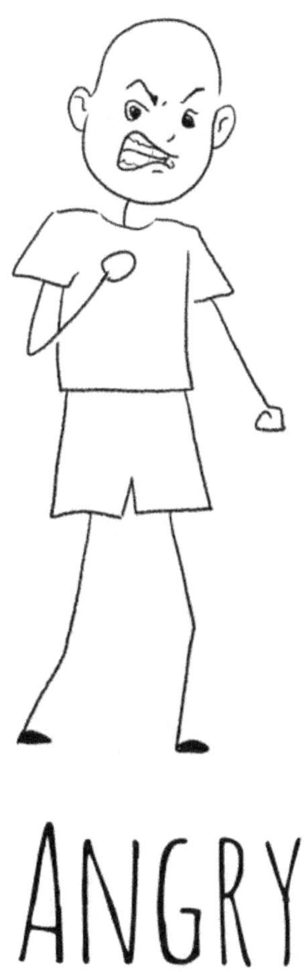

ANGRY

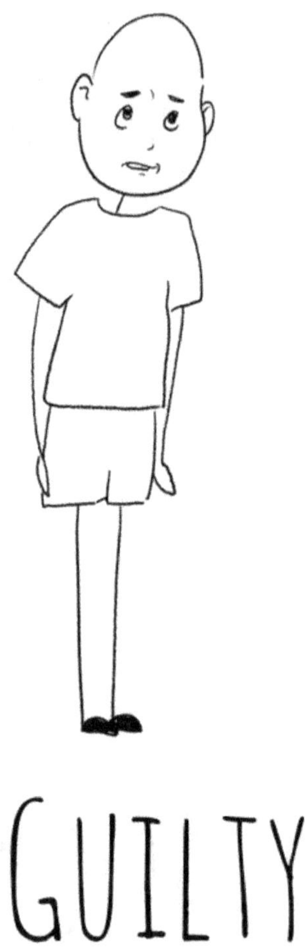

GUILTY

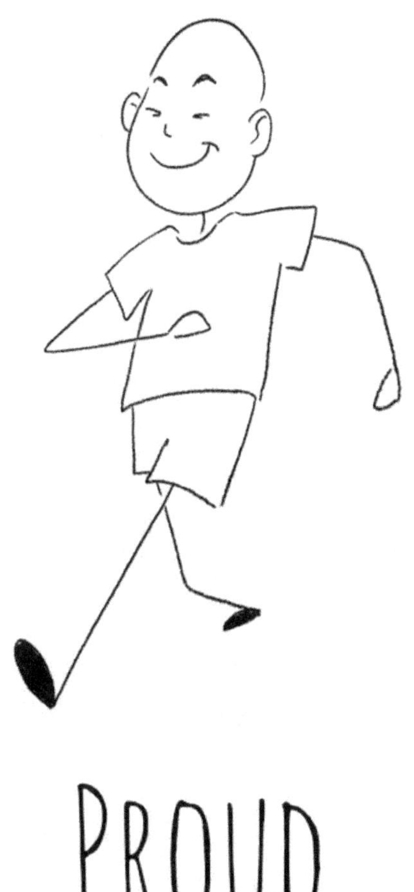

PROUD

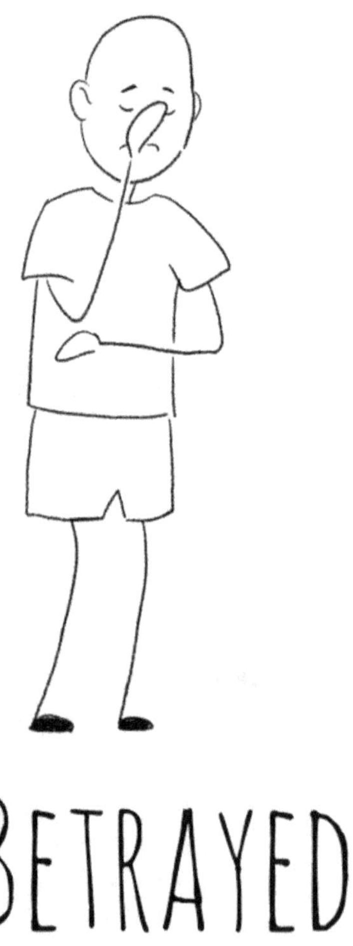

BETRAYED

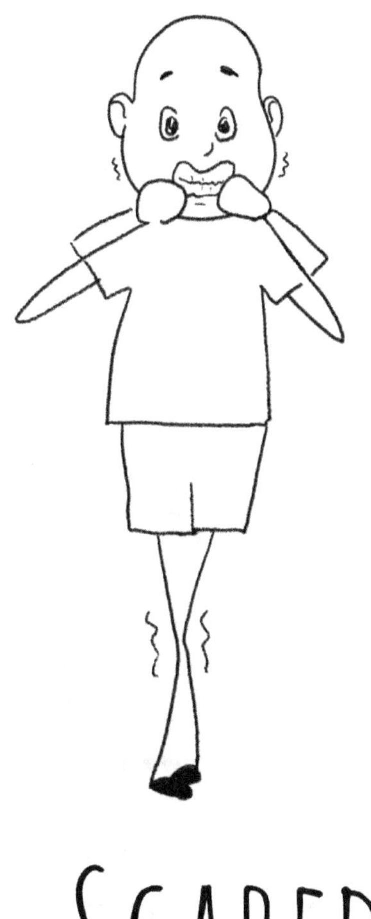

SCARED

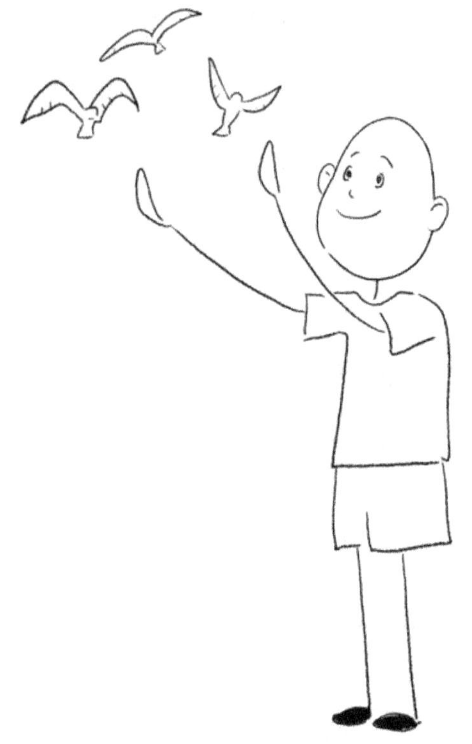

FORGIVENESS

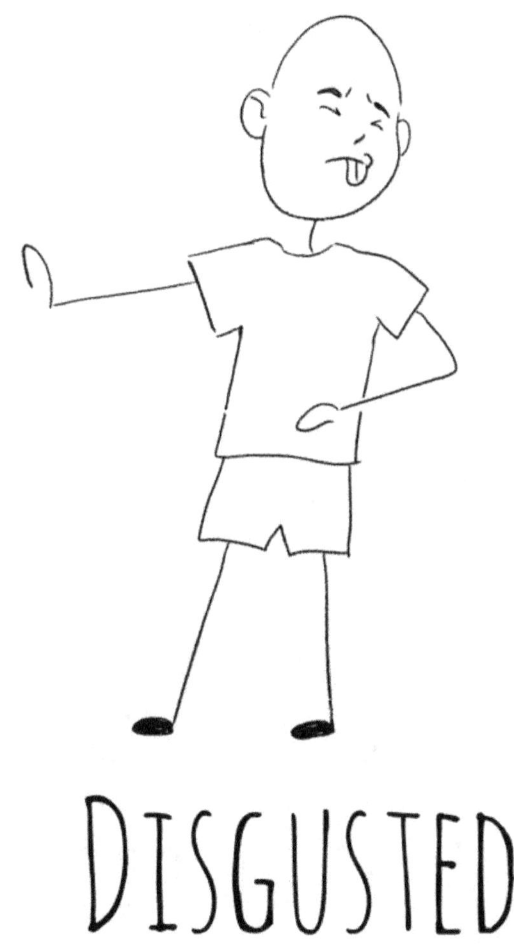

DISGUSTED

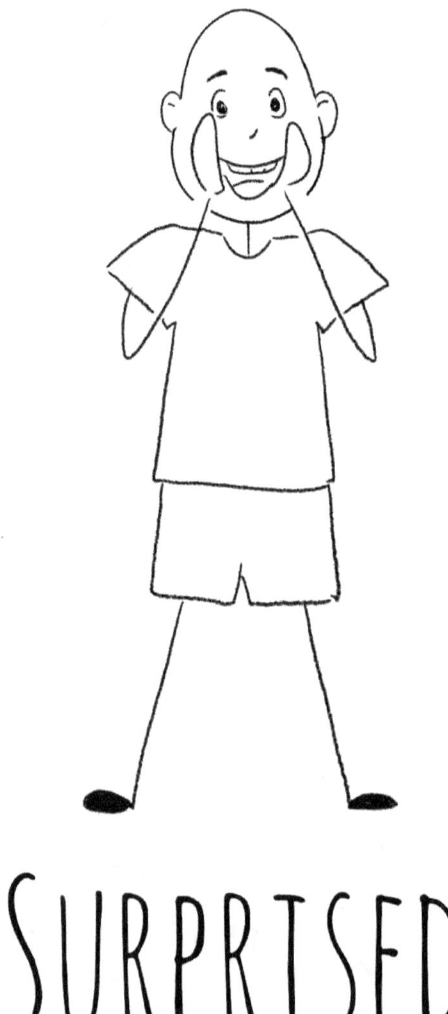

SURPRISED

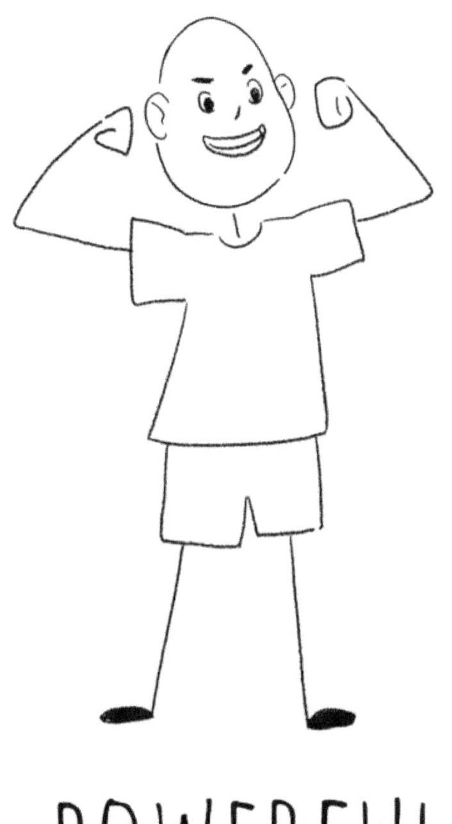

POWERFUL

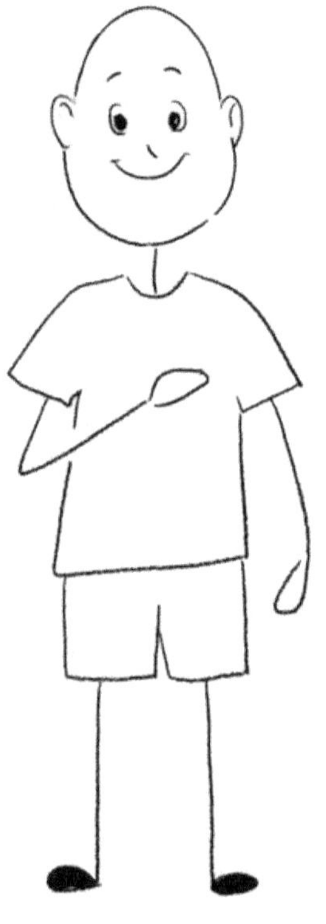

UNDERSTOOD

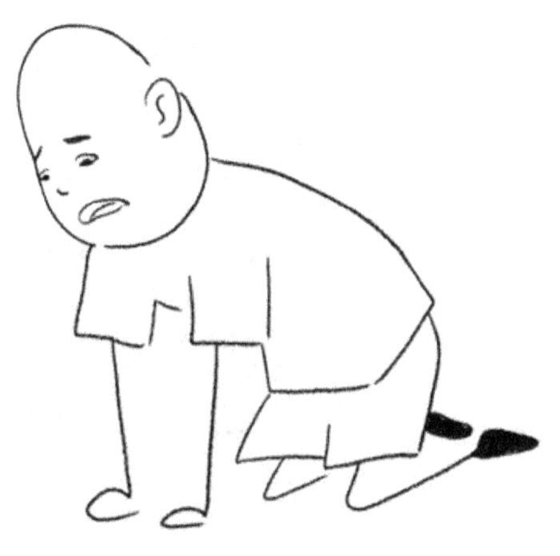

HOPELESS

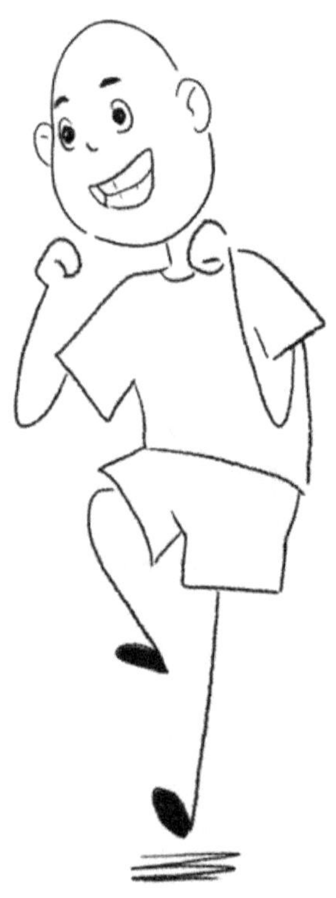

EAGER

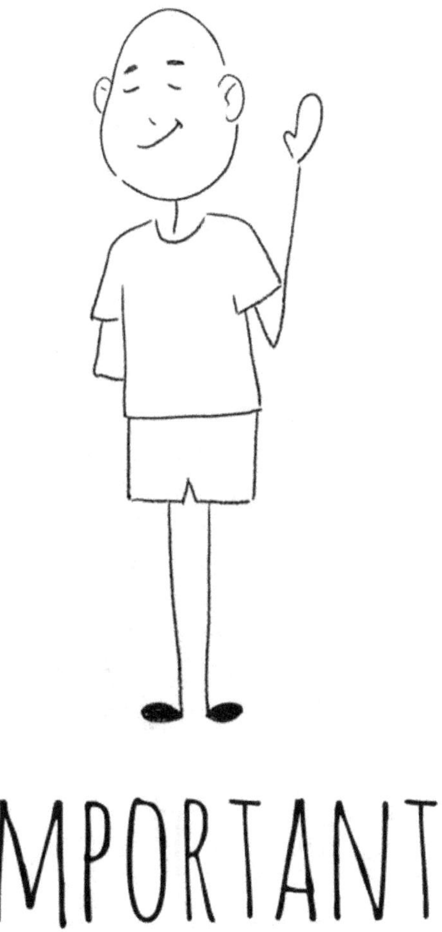

IMPORTANT

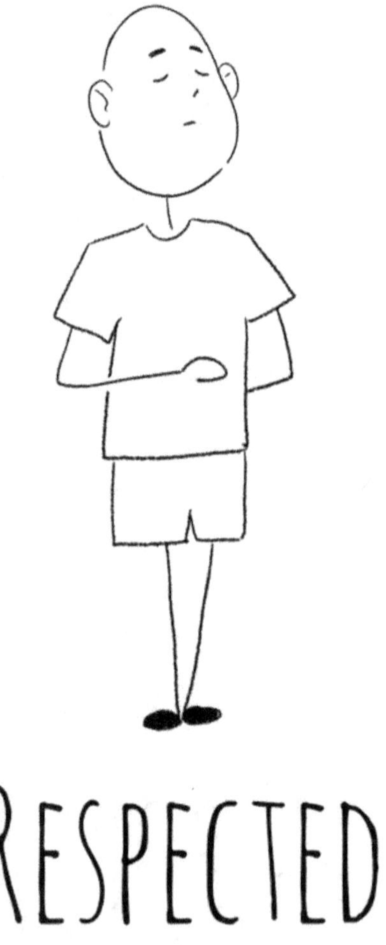

RESPECTED

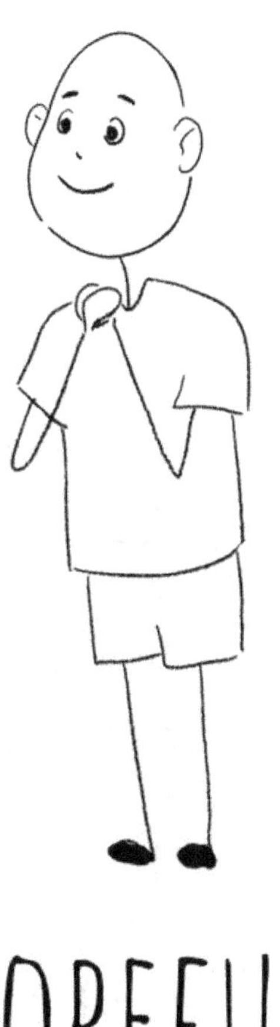

HOPEFUL

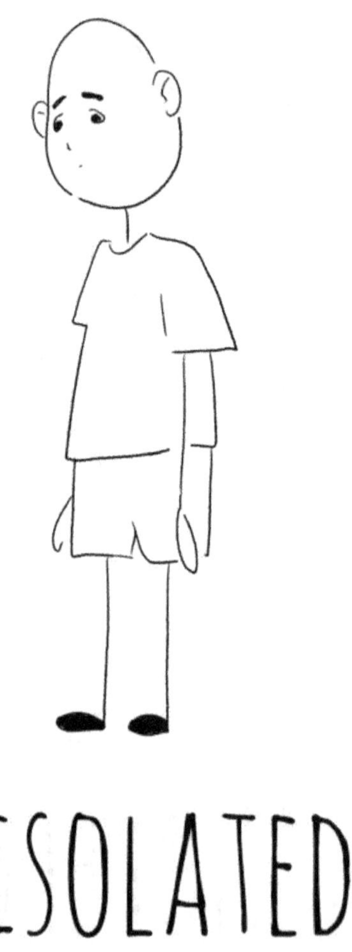

ISOLATED

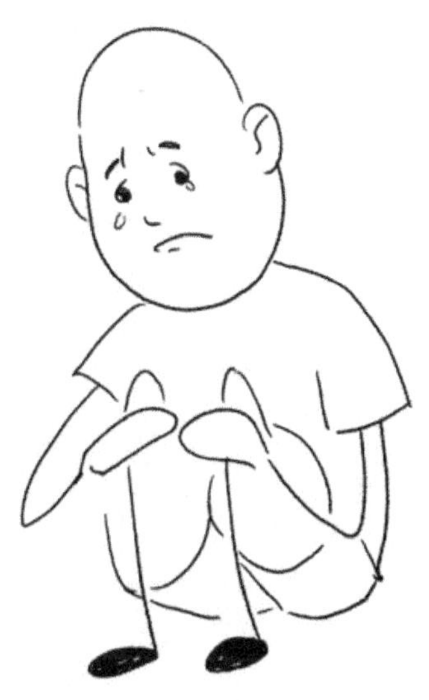

REJECTED

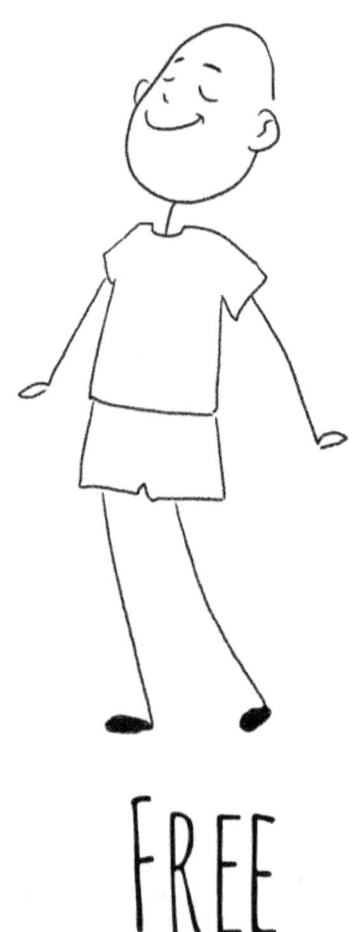

FREE

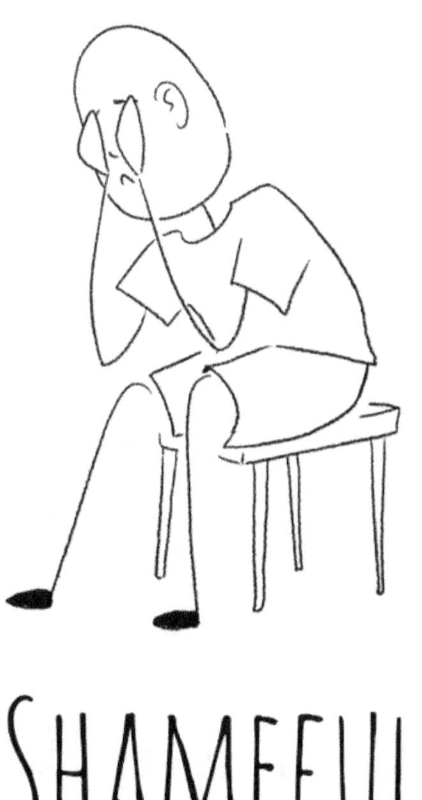

SHAMEFUL

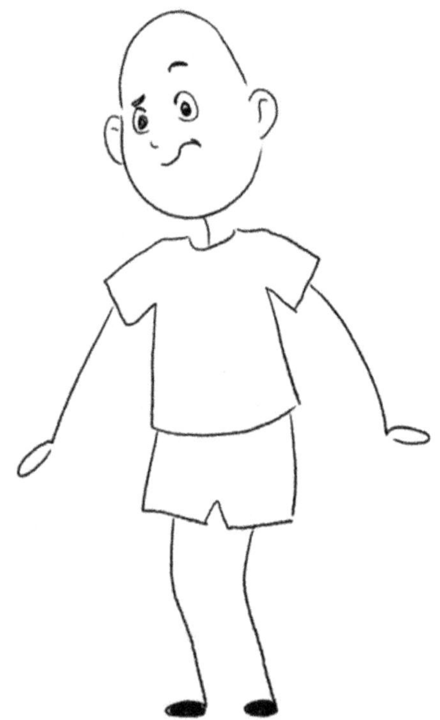

CONFUSED

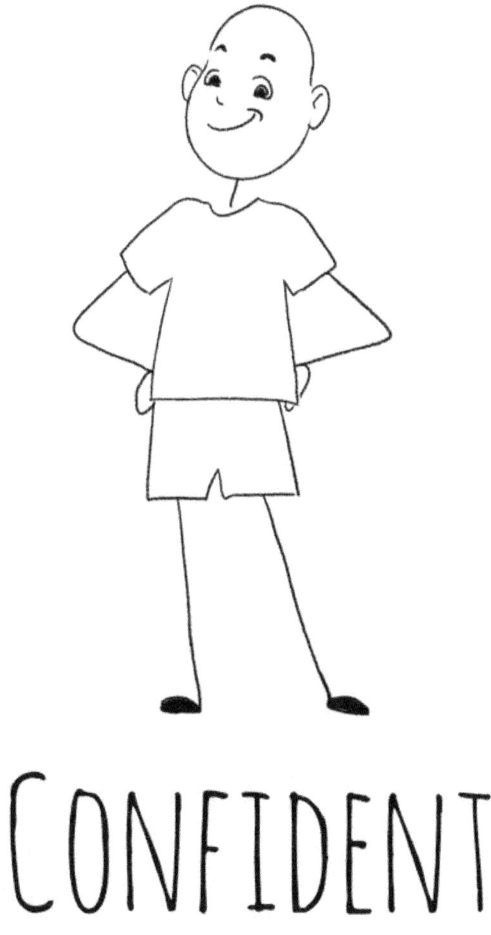

CONFIDENT

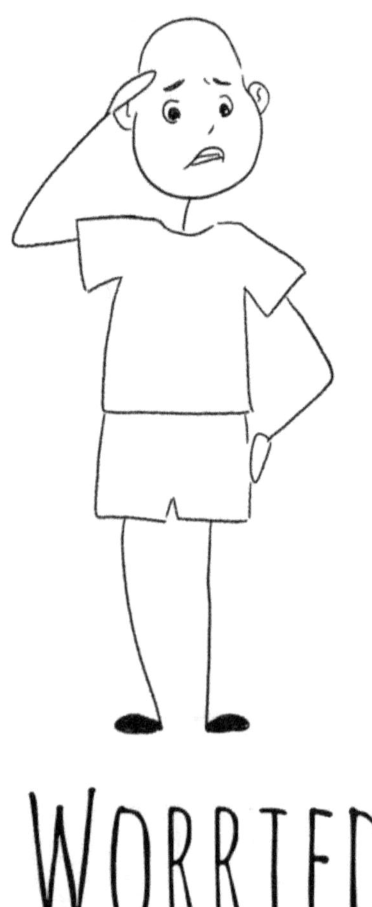

WORRIED

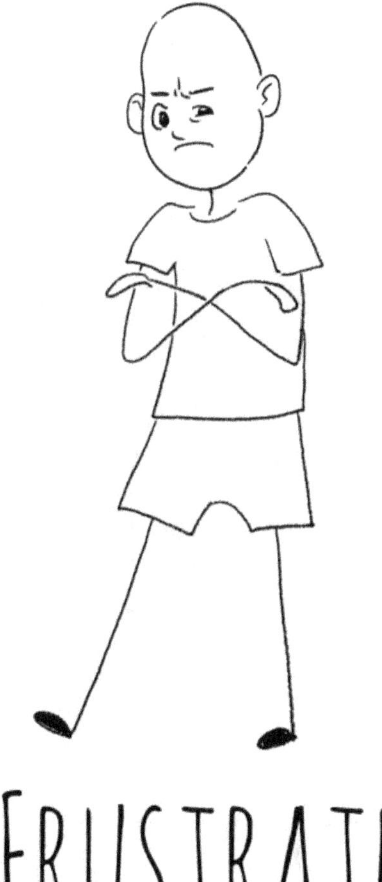

FRUSTRATED

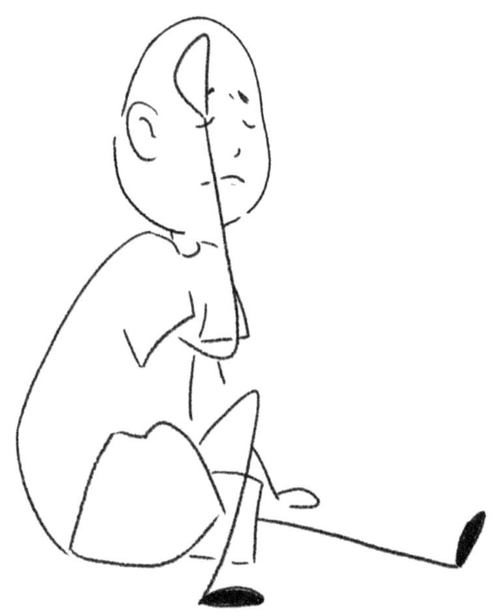

INSIGNIFICANT

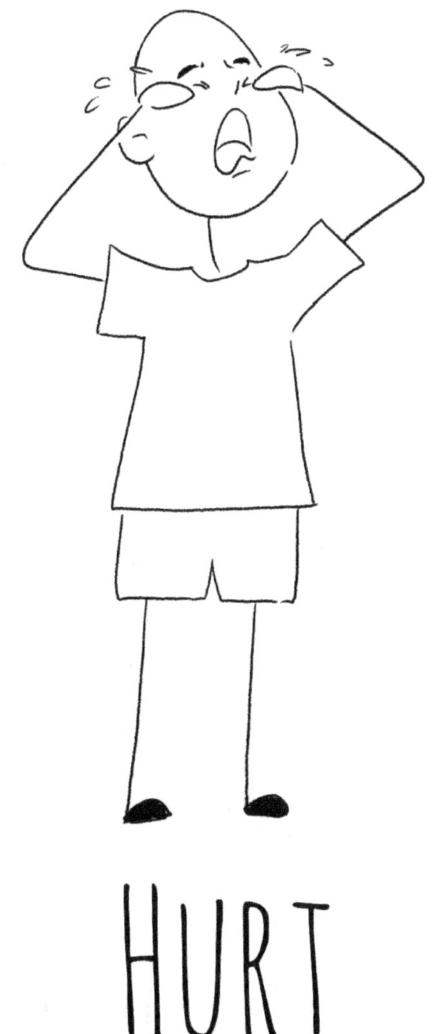

HURT

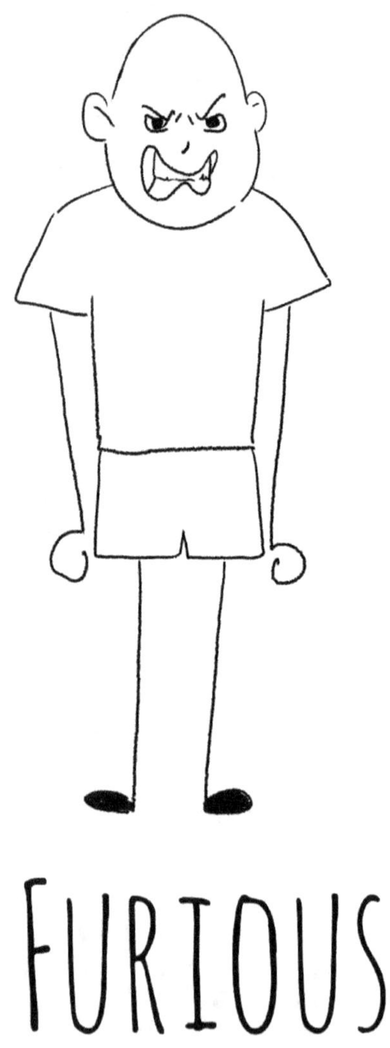

FURIOUS

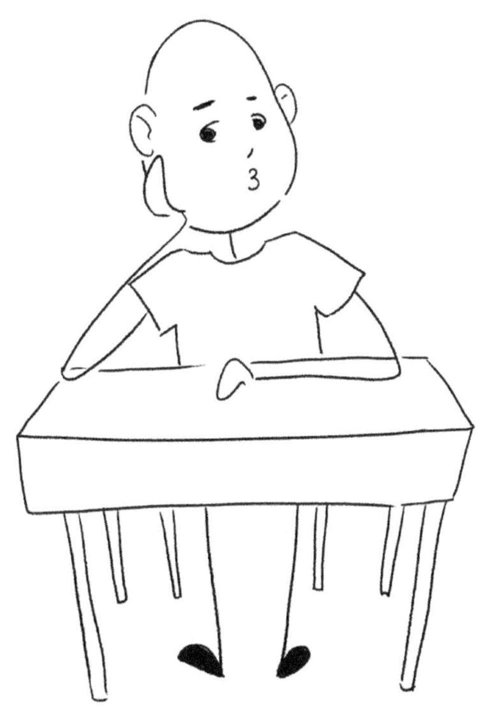

BORED

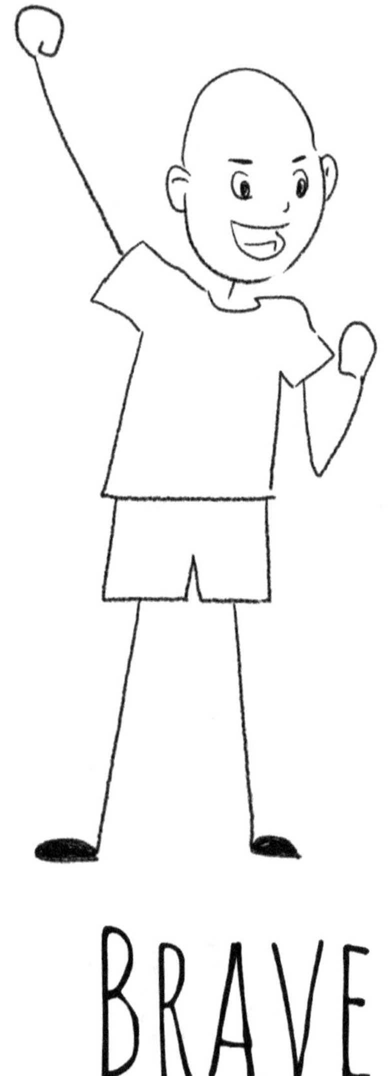

BRAVE

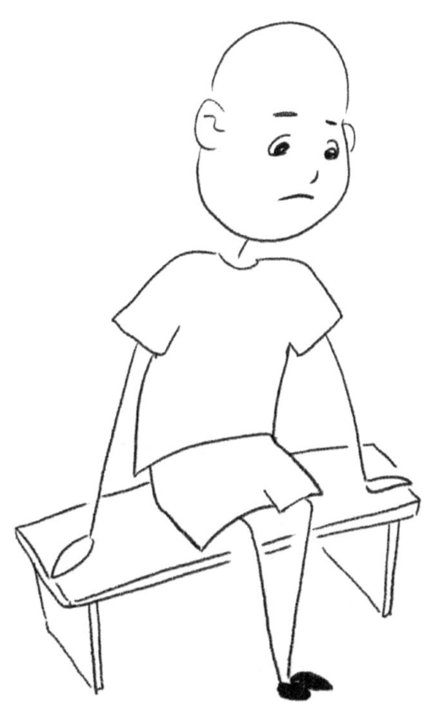

LONELY

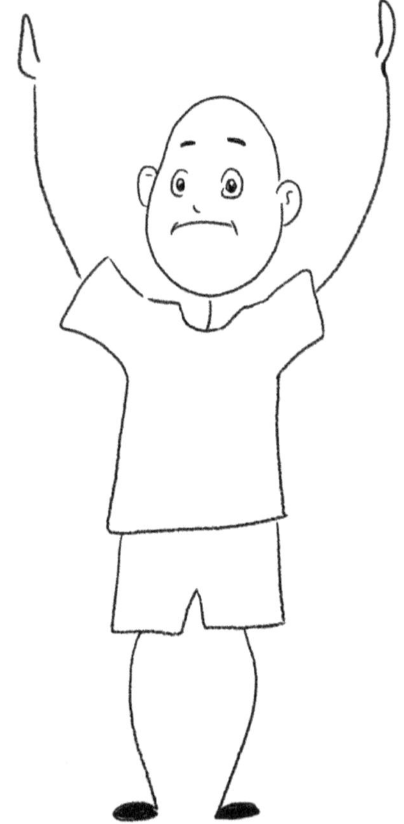

OVERWHELMED

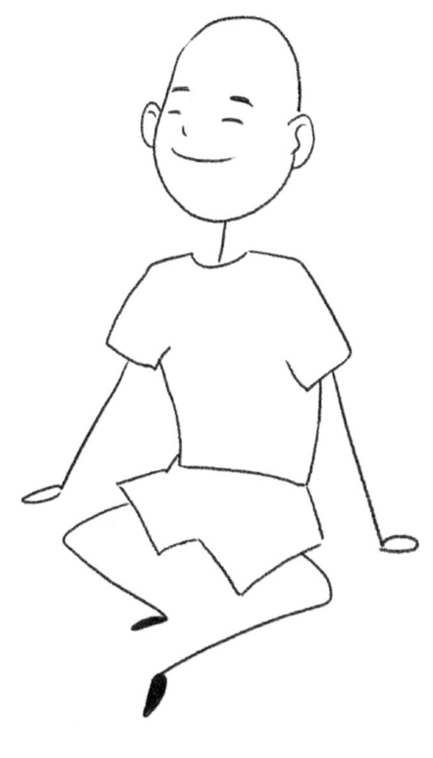

PEACEFUL